The Hemorrhoids Handbook

By Thorsten Hawk

Content

Hemorrhoids, what's that?

Hemorrhoids are also called haemorrides, which comes from ancient Greek and means "to flow blood". This is an ancient term for it. Hemorrhoids are vascular cushions (arteriovenous). They are ring-shaped and are located under the rectal mucosa. They are used for fine closure of the anus.

Thus, the hemorrhoids form a vascular cushion at the anus which is traversed by many veins. They are just above the inner sphincter. In this way, they support the sphincter muscle in its maintenance and serve for intestinal continence. No stool can ever escape uncontrolled through them.

We have two sphincters and the inner one holds the receptors inside the mucous membrane, which then trigger the urge to defecate. When we have a certain amount of stool in our rectum, the urge to defecate is triggered. The outer sphincters then consciously induce or suppress the bowel movement.

Why do hemorrhoids exist?

Hemorrhoids - what is that, many ask themselves. It is important to be able to recognize hemorrhoids. The sphincter muscle alone is often not able to close the intestine effectively from the outside. For the so-called "fine continence" our body needs the hemorrhoids. When they fill with blood, they swell. They then increasingly seal the bowel outlet. If you have a bowel movement, this causes the blood to drain off and the vascular cushion to retract so that the excrement can also pass through. The varicose vein-like and nodular swellings are therefore an expansion of the cavernous body (vascular cushion).

Hemorrhoids causes?

The causes of the plexus hemorrhoidal often include inflammation of the surrounding tissue. These swellings cause hemorrhoids to be gradually pushed out of the anus. Chronic constipation is one of the main causes of hemorrhoids. They can be caused by a lack of exercise, overweight and incorrect nutrition. However, many people also suffer from a weakness of the vascular walls.

Women also often have problems with this after pregnancy.

If you press too hard on the toilet, you will also get hemorrhoids in the long run. Chronic constipation can also be a cause. Work involving heavy lifting also causes hemorrhoids in the long term. Carrying heavy loads causes pressure on the abdomen and thus on the intestinal area.

Frequent diarrhea is also considered a cause of hemorrhoids. Liquid stool causes inflammation to develop quickly, which then triggers the problem. During pregnancy, the baby presses on the womb and thus on the rectum, which is one of the reasons for this cause.

Obesity in general can also cause a reduced blood flow and thus trigger hemorrhoids. The blood circulation in the intestine is blocked by the overweight and thus the outflow of blood from the vascular pads is inhibited.

Why do hemorrhoids develop?

Hemorrhoids occur because many people also have bad stool habits. As a result, more and wrong and too violently pressed during bowel movement. This causes the formation of hemorrhoids. Through the violent pressing a lot of blood is pressed into the erectile tissue. This in turn prevents the blood from draining away. The cavernous bodies are then not pushed to the side as desired, but outwards. This causes hemorrhoids. Chronic constipation also causes people to suffer. People who eat a low-fiber diet, have little exercise and drink too little, risk developing hemorrhoids if they press hard.

Hemorrhoids after birth and hemorrhoids in pregnancy often affect women. This is the case in half of all expectant mothers. Women who have already had problems before are particularly affected. During pregnancy and after giving birth the problems often worsen.

The pregnancy hormones deliberately set the body to "wide" and "soft". This then affects the skin, the connective tissue, the vessels, the pelvic floor and everything else. This also affects the vessels in the rectum. The appearance of hemorrhoids varies depending on how severely the woman is affected. In addition, during pregnancy one often suffers from a lack of exercise, which in turn makes the intestine even slower. Then, at the latest, comes the question: What helps against hemorrhoids?

For many women this is an unpleasant and again pressing issue during pregnancy and before birth. It is important to recognize hemorrhoids at the anus quickly in order to be able to act. Those that have already come out can be palpated and felt. Hemorrhoids - what helps immediately? Fighting constipation is an important way for expectant mothers.

A fiber-rich diet is crucial. Drinking plenty of water is also important. Natural yoghurt, a tablespoon of linseed or flea seed is valuable. Always drink a large glass of water with it and eat dried fruit. Prune juice also helps pregnant women to avoid this condition. It is important not to use laxatives, as this can worsen intestinal sluggishness in the long-term during pregnancy but also in general.
However, an enema (a rectal lavage) can be useful after the birth. It is also important for expectant mothers to know that iron tablets basically cause a rather solid stool. They can therefore cause constipation and therefore lead to hemorrhoids.

Therefore, other types of iron replacement, such as a herbal blood juice, are more sensible. In addition, it is also recommended that pregnant women who are healthy and fit should exercise a lot. A hemorrhoid cushion is useful for jobs where you have to sit for long periods.

Hemorrhoid symptoms?

Hemorrhoids bleed or itch, many people know that, a hemorrhoid cream can help here, but what are the symptoms exactly? In the beginning they usually cause little discomfort, the first signs are usually traces of very light blood from the stool or underwear. Many also notice it when going to the toilet on toilet paper. Then there is usually a burning sensation. Later, they may also itch.

If the vascular cushions of the hemorrhoids then become larger and larger, then the complaints also increase. The itching and burning become worse in the anal area. Often it is a weeping anus and a re-lubrication of stool, which is then disturbing. The bright red blood deposits on the stool are unpleasant and frightening for many people affected. The blood can also be seen on toilet paper. Often there is also a feeling that the bowel could not be emptied completely.

An unpleasant feeling of pressure that many complain about. Many of those affected always have several symptoms together and find this very unpleasant. These complaints and symptoms can considerably impair the general well-being. In any case, the symptoms are manifold and can range from painless bleeding to severe itching or annoying burning. Weeping and inflammation of the anus follow and the feeling of incomplete bowel movement.

The smearing of stools is considered particularly unpleasant. A persistent urge to defecate with an unpleasant feeling of pressure or pain in the anal region also occurs. Here it must be clarified whether another serious illness is present. The proctologist is the doctor of choice in this case.

Why do hemorrhoids itch?

Hemorrhoids itch, it is well known, but why is this so? The proctological cause of the itching is the constantly humid environment. As a result, the skin is very irritated and the itching tends to occur. By the way, hemorrhoids are generally favored by gastro-intestinal diseases. These also include the autoimmune diseases ulcerative colitis or Crohn's disease. These can generally cause long-lasting diarrhea and thus trigger hemorrhoids. Hemorrhoids what helps immediately one asks oneself when the itching becomes unbearable. Then a hemorrhoid ointment is a good decision, it relieves the itching quickly and in a pleasant, simple way. Within the hemorrhoid stages, the itching usually occurs at the beginning.

Why do hemorrhoids bleed?

The topic of hemorrhoids is often still a taboo subject, with one in three people suffering from this disease. When the vascular cushions cause bleeding during bowel movements, they become a burden. The sight of bleeding hemorrhoids is usually shocking, but it is usually harmless. The symptoms must nevertheless be taken very seriously. There can be different causes behind them. It is a fact that not only hemorrhoids can cause bleeding in the anal area. There are several causes for this. These can also include diseases of the lower, middle and upper digestive tract. A gastrointestinal ulcer, for example, can cause bleeding. Irritated stomach lining or liver disease can also cause bleeding. Also, certain drugs or frequent vomiting. Stomach cancer can also cause bleeding. It is therefore important to see a doctor if the bleeding is unclear and have it checked.

The cause of hemorrhoids bleeding is usually due to a progression of the disease. In hemorrhoidal disease with a severity of four or three, these vascular cushions can then protrude from the rectum. The friction and itching can then cause bleeding. Excessive pressing during bowel movement also triggers this. The internal hemorrhoids usually do not cause bleeding in the stool.

The outer anal canal can be blocked by hemorrhoids. They then often burst due to the strong pressing during defecation. They can also start to bleed if they are blocked. Then the veins simply do not have time for the blood to drain off inside the vessels. The affected person then sees the blood in the stool or on the toilet paper or in the toilet. If the bleeding becomes heavier or lasts longer, one should urgently consult a doctor.

Bleeding during defecation is usually not dangerous if the blood is light red to pink in color. Nevertheless, they should never be taken lightly. If the blood is black or dark and there is pain, then it may be a serious gastrointestinal disease and a visit to the doctor is essential. If hemorrhoids have leaked, then an incarceration may occur. This is the case when the erectile tissue is trapped (anal canal). Then the blood in the vessels becomes congested and the blood flow is then slowed down. In severe cases this can trigger a thrombosis. People who suffer from hemorrhoids that bleed heavily and often bleed can even suffer from anemia. The symptoms of this are dizziness and tiredness. As a rule, however, bleeding during bowel movements is not dangerous. For safety reasons, however, one should consult a proctologist.

Tip: Special ointments and creams are suitable for stopping light bleeding. These then contract the blood vessels. Aloe vera can also help here and accelerate the healing of wounds. In general, moist toilet paper is gentler than the classic one. It does not rub against the hemorrhoids and you should rather dab than wipe. Moist toilet paper cleans the anus more thoroughly and thus the risk of infection is minimized.

The doctor will then make a detailed diagnosis of bleeding hemorrhoids. The question comes up whether blood-thinning medication should be taken. Also, a pathological bleeding tendency must be clarified. Signs of this would be frequent nosebleeds or frequently occurring bruises. Ointments with "astringents" are used here. These are hemostatic agents that have an anti-inflammatory and antibacterial effect at the same time. Sitting baths and suppositories can also help. These then relieve the hemorrhoidal problem.

If hemorrhoids bleed, it is usually during bowel movements. It can also be triggered by external stimuli.

As a rule, the body can regulate the healing of wounds by itself. When the hemorrhoids are gone, there is no more bleeding. However, if regular bleeding occurs, it must be clarified by a doctor. It is also important to make sure that a softer stool prevails. A diet rich in fiber is important in this case. A sufficient fluid intake should also be taken into account.

first degree hemorrhoids

The studies show that 70 percent of adults over 30 years of age have hemorrhoids of varying degrees and stages. However, many people have hardly any symptoms. A distinction is therefore made between hemorrhoids with and hemorrhoids without complaints and symptoms. At the 1st degree the hemorrhoids are not visible at all. The doctor or the patient cannot yet feel them. They cause only minimal symptoms. They can usually be treated with over-the-counter creams, ointments and medicines. A change in everyday life can help here. At the 1st degree the vascular cushions are only slightly enlarged. They can then be identified by colonoscopy. At the first degree, the patient still has no symptoms when pressing. Occasionally light red, minimal traces of blood can be found on the toilet paper. The anus itches sometimes.

Second-degree hemorrhoids

The 2nd degree hemorrhoids appear temporarily after bowel movements. They can also appear during stress. Here, for example, it is possible that the hemorrhoidal nodes first pull outwards during pressing. Then they usually retract again. In most cases the enlargements are then clearly visible and palpable from the outside and the affected person has a foreign body sensation that is unpleasant.

Third degree hemorrhoids

In severity 3, the hemorrhoids have definitely come out and cannot be pushed back easily. Nor do they automatically go back after pressing. It is recommended to push them back gently at the clean anus. There is also usually inflammation at degree 3. Swelling is also present here. The patient with degree 3 usually has severe pain during bowel movement. In addition, continuous itching and mucous membrane secretions plague the patient.

Fourth degree hemorrhoids

Anyone suffering from fourth degree hemorrhoids has a constant prolapse. The symptoms become severe and massive inflammation occurs. It is essential to find a solution with the proctologist. Surgical intervention is often the case. At the fourth degree, incontinence can also occur.

Hemorrhoid therapy?

The question about the treatment of hemorrhoids is easily answered: There is the conservative therapy and the surgical therapy. The conservative therapies can be used for degree 1 and 2. Surgical therapy is usually applied at degree 3 and 4.

In conservative therapy there are ointments and suppositories for treatment. However, these should not be used indefinitely, but only for a short time. They can relieve the acute symptoms and ease the pain. A fundamental solution to the hemorrhoidal problem is usually not possible. A general tip for people who want additional support is to practice precise, careful but not excessive anal hygiene. This would be mainly water and no soap additives. A bowel regulation of hard bowel movements is also important. Long periods of sitting and strong pressing are negative. Sclerotherapy is common in conservative therapy for degree 1 and 2. This is a sclerotherapy of the hemorrhoids. This reduces the hemorrhoid cushion. Then it can retract into the rectum. There is an alternative method to sclerotherapy. This is the rubber band ligature. This is becoming more and more popular. Here the hemorrhoids are first sucked in. Then they are virtually tied off with sterile rubber bands. After a few days already, the constricted tissue is rejected. This happens by itself. With hemorrhoids with the 2nd and 3rd degree this application can take place.

Surgical therapy should be considered for patients who have the 3rd or 4th degree of hemorrhoids. There are various surgical procedures to carefully remove the hemorrhoids including the blood vessels. The so-called stacker method is a new procedure in this area. It is just as successful as the usual surgical procedures during an operation, but the patient has some advantages. In a so-called stacker operation, an instrument is first inserted into the anus. Then the hemorrhoids are maneuvered into a "tissue cuff" that is about one centimeter wide. The hemorrhoids can then be operated out and the intestinal wall is then sutured together with metal clips. Compared to the usual operations, the patient has less pain after the procedure. The duration of the hospital stay is also reduced.

It is important to know that neither the surgical therapies nor the conservative therapies guarantee a lasting and final success of the therapy. Nevertheless, sometimes hemorrhoids reappear after a few years and lead to complaints. A new treatment is necessary in this case.

What helps immediately?

For acute complaints of degree 1 and 2, cold helps as an immediate remedy. Here you can either press the classic toilet paper with ice-cold water against the hemorrhoids or put a small ice bag in a washcloth. Then this is pressed against the anal area for a few minutes, maximum ten minutes. The pressing must be gentle. The cold causes all blood vessels to contract again and bleeding is also prevented.

Linseed is a perfect household remedy for hemorrhoids. Taken with plenty of liquid it not only promotes healthy digestion, but the mucilage also promotes a pleasant, soft bowel movement. Sitting baths with chamomile or anti-inflammatory tanning agents are also recommended. This includes oak bark. This helps against itching and pain. Basically, suppositories and ointments with witch hazel and chamomile are suitable as household remedies. Jojoba wax is also a suitable household remedy for externally visible and palpable hemorrhoids. They can be cared for with it and at degree 1 and 2 they also disappear with care.

An oak bark hip bath contains tanning agents that have an astringent effect. The diseased tissue thus contracts again. Itching and weeping can also be relieved in this way. For this purpose, a handful of oak bark is first cooked on a low flame at the stove for a quarter of an hour from the pharmacy. Then you leave it for a while and you have a special sitz bath that can be hung in the toilet. Thus, one does not need a chair. The strong essence of the oak bark extract helps the vessel cushions to contract again.

Which cream helps?

The commercially available creams against hemorrhoids usually relieve the itching and pain. There are anti-inflammatory variants. In addition to panthenol and herbal active ingredients, they also contain zinc and witch hazel or aloe vera. But creams with cortisone are also available. For stronger pain and severe itching and 2nd and 3rd degree hemorrhoids these stronger creams are suitable.

As a general rule, creams and ointments can help with mild complaints such as itching and swelling. The anal tampons, suppositories and a mullein insert with suppositories can also help, as can sitz baths from the pharmacy. All creams contain anti-inflammatory and local anesthetics. Vasoconstricting agents are also included. The pharmacist will be happy to advise you which cream is best for you. They relieve the symptoms in the short term, but cannot be used as a permanent therapy. The actual cause is not eliminated by creams.

Hemorrhoid suppositories?

For hemorrhoids that are also internal, suppositories that also contain analgesic and anti-inflammatory agents are particularly suitable. They can be used in combination with the cream of the same active ingredient or separately. They reduce swelling and alleviate the worst symptoms such as itching and inflammation. The braids also act as a lubricant to reduce hemorrhoids in the long term. The inflammation and itching usually disappears quickly. The normal function of the anal mucosa is supported. There are also suppositories in a set with the cream and depending on the severity of the problem, a variant with painkillers and cortisone should be chosen. The proctologist helps here and writes the prescription for the prescription drugs.

Seat cushion?

With 3rd and 4th degree hemorrhoids, many patients choose a seat cushion. This hemorrhoid cushion can relieve the pain when sitting. The affected region is thus relieved and the acute complaints are reduced. Such seat cushions are also recommended after hemorrhoid surgery. Because especially after the operation the patient often has pain when sitting. The seat cushion is a seat ring that gently relieves the affected anal region.

Which doctor?

Many people wonder which doctor is responsible for hemorrhoids. The doctor for hemorrhoids is the proctologist. A treatment of diseased hemorrhoids is also often performed by a surgeon. However, the doctor who is basically specialized in the anus is the proctologist. However, nobody needs to be afraid, the operation is not always performed in the same way. Sclerosing hemorrhoids is also a possibility that can usually be done on an outpatient basis. The hemorrhoid medication will also help locally with mild forms. Hemorrhoids to which doctor is therefore quickly answered. If the degree is severe, the hemorrhoids must be removed. Hemorrhoid home remedy or hemorrhoid surgery, the proctologist will certainly answer the question competently.

Hemorrhoid surgery?

If surgery is necessary for degree 3 and 4, many patients want to know the details. If the hemorrhoids become larger and larger, the symptoms such as itching, burning, weeping and pain become much stronger and the pressure of suffering increases. Everyday life is made more difficult by the signs of the disease and sitting can be extremely painful. The bowel movement also hurts and then surgical treatment is recommended.

Normally, the vascular cushions on the rectum do not cause any problems, but surgery is necessary if the symptoms greatly interfere with everyday life. The symptoms of weeping, burning, itching and pain are then called hemorrhoidal disorders in the specialist Jargon. Surgical removal of the troublesome hemorrhoids is called a hemorrhoidectomy. The cause of such hemorrhoids can be anal eczema, a rectum prolapse, an anal thrombosis or a meniscus. In most cases, however, surgery is not common until the final stage. In degree 3 and 4 the hemorrhoids are located outside (anus) and cannot be treated as easily with ointments and creams or suppositories. The proctologist advises the affected person exactly whether and which surgery is necessary.

The medical treatment measures that can be carried out on an outpatient and inpatient basis include obliteration, rubber band ligation, the THD method, hemorrhoidectomy, surgery according to Longo and laser radiation. The patient is first informed about all treatment options. As a rule, general anesthesia takes place during a hemorrhoid operation. Bleeding can always occur during an operation, as the cushion of blood vessels is removed with a scalpel. This risk of bleeding remains even after the operation, which is why long-term observation is necessary. Many patients are allowed to go home immediately after the operation, but a stay of three to four days after the operation is usual. After a rubber band ligation, some patients are allowed to leave the hospital or practice immediately after the operation. Laser treatments also usually do not require a longer stay.

Cauterize or remove?

The proctologist advises the patient whether obliteration or removal is appropriate. The basic measures, such as a healthy diet, a lot of exercise and good anal hygiene must always be accompanied. Cauterization is one of the very first treatment methods suggested by the proctologist.

This method belongs to the conservative treatment methods.

During the obliteration, a solution is injected into the node of the hemorrhoids with a proctoscope, which is an examination instrument especially for the anal canal. In this way the blood supply is first of all throttled. The vessel cushions then lose volume. This procedure of sclerotherapy is usually carried out on an outpatient basis; an inpatient stay is not necessary. The sclerotherapy can be performed in the proctological practice and the patient can go home immediately after the treatment.

How long does healing take?

After hemorrhoid surgery, the patient should expect a recovery period of two to four weeks. Although the operation is not a major procedure, a little rest and observation is important. The higher the degree of the disease, the longer the recovery usually takes. With degree 3 and 4, the hemorrhoids do not recede by themselves, and lacing off with a rubber band ligature or desertification are important. Here, several weeks of healing time must be expected. At degree 1 and 2 it usually takes two to three weeks until the hemorrhoids have healed again.

During surgery, the techniques are more and more innovative and gentle, and therefore there are usually no complications. Post-bleeding is rare and therefore healing takes two to four weeks. The suture holds well and the scar rarely leaks. Anyone who has pain after the operation must take painkillers for a while. As a rule, a grace period of two to four weeks must be observed. After one month at the latest, patients usually feel well again. As a rule, a sick note of two to four weeks is required. With degree 1 and 2 you do not drop out of the working life and can help even with the conservative creams and ointments.

Hemorrhoid diet

Nutrition is particularly important for long-term success and the prevention of hemorrhoids. It should be optimized so that the bowel movement is not too hard or too thin in a natural way. The intestine must be kept healthy. For this purpose, a diet rich in fiber and low in fat is sensible. It should not be too spicy, because hot spices irritate the intestine. Regular emptying of the bowel is the goal. The stool should be softly shaped, but also not too thin. This prevents irritation of the anal mucosa from the outset.

Regular drinking is also important. The daily amount of fluid should be at least two to three liters. Water is the best here; unsweetened herbal tea is also good. In any case, the most important thing for hemorrhoids is a healthy diet and drinking a lot. Both orthodox medicine and natural medicine see it that way. Because through a regular digestion the basis can be created that a hemorrhoidal disease does not exist at all. To avoid and prevent this, a healthy, wholesome and vitamin-rich diet is recommended. It should contain a lot of fiber in the form of whole meal products. The old cereals such as millet, amaranth and quinoa, which are also gluten-free, are also good for a healthy intestine. Vegetables and fruit should be on the regular menu. In addition, milk products are excellent for producing a healthy digestion in the long term because of their lactic acidity. The stool should be kept soft and then there is not much pressing to do. This is the best prevention against hemorrhoids.

It is particularly important to avoid the stuffing food and beverages. This includes above all chocolate, which not only has many calories but also clogs. Also, coffee and cola should be avoided or reduced. Black tea also belongs to the stuffing foods. It is also important to ensure that white flour products are excluded from the menu. Sweets should also be left out. Dried fruit is a suitable alternative. Spicy spices such as chili or curry should also be reduced. The tender anal mucosa suffers from this and can be irritated.

What can I eat?

A fresh grain muesli or whole meal bread is suitable for breakfast. Some fruit and vegetables provide the necessary fiber and vitamins. Raw vegetable salads are also an ideal snack or main meal in a healthy, wholesome diet. Dairy products such as buttermilk, quark, yoghurt and cheese in moderation are important. Fresh fruit is suitable for dessert. Plenty of water and herbal or fruit teas provide the necessary liquid.

If an affected person does not achieve success despite an optimized and wholesome diet rich in fiber and does not have regular digestion, he or she should talk to the doctor or pharmacist about it. Anyone suffering from chronic constipation makes the situation worse. Some intestinal bacteria may be missing and can be supplied. Probiotic agents also help. Laxatives are not advisable, as they lead to sluggishness in the bowel in the long run. The complaints will only get worse.

Hemorrhoid prophylaxis?

A healthy diet is part of the best prevention. However, sufficient exercise should also be planned for hemorrhoids. Those who work in sedentary jobs must get a fitness app or a fitness watch or other tricks and run regularly. Especially endurance sports or regular running are important to ensure that the body has enough exercise. Gentle but continuous movement is important. Sports and habits play a major role in everyday life.

Ideal sports include running, hiking, gymnastics, swimming or more strenuous sports such as tennis, jumping, jogging or a team sport. Comfort is negative and this is often only the beginning of suffering. It is important to change your habits and to plan for additional exercise.

The best way to prevent this is to learn to do so. Walking the stairs instead of using the elevator is a start. Doing little shopping and errands on foot and leaving the car at home can help enormously in the long run.

Anal hygiene is also part of prevention. The important thing is never to wipe, but always to dab. A damp toilet paper is better than a dry one.

If you simply moisten your dry toilet paper under the tap, you save twice as much money, and there are also no harmful fragrances. Lukewarm water is pleasant when cleaning the anus. There are also special water sprayers that help to keep the anus thoroughly clean. A disposable washcloth also helps to keep the anus clean.

Careful dabbing, no Scratch or rubbing, is ideal for perfect anal hygiene. Those who use special anal templates can also satisfy their need for cleanliness.

Legal notice:

I am not a doctor!

It is expressly pointed out that the tips, information, products and instructions presented here in no way replace a visit to the doctor.

This is not medical advice.

The information and texts presented here are not an invitation to self-diagnosis.

 All texts and information are for informal purposes only. They have been carefully researched and checked, but no liability is accepted for the accuracy of all information.

Follow the tips at your own risk. Always consult your attending physician if you have health questions or complaints.

Imprint

© 2020 Randy Bolz

Sterndamm 17

12487 Berlin

Edition (1)

Cover design, Illustration: Randy Bolz
Editing, Proofreading: Randy Bolz
Translation: Randy Bolz
Publisher: Randy Bolz
Printers: Amazon Europe in Luxembourg